A Practical Guide to Posttraumatic Stress Disorder (PTSD)

Kristi Kanel

California State University, Fullerton

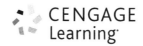

CENGAGE
Learning

Australia • Brazil • Mexico • Singapore • United Kingdom • United States

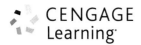

ISBN: 978-1-305-40096-2

Cengage Learning
20 Channel Center Street
Boston, MA 02210
USA

Cengage Learning is a leading provider of customized learning solutions with office locations around the globe, including Singapore, the United Kingdom, Australia, Mexico, Brazil, and Japan. Locate your local office at: **www.cengage.com/global**.

Cengage Learning products are represented in Canada by Nelson Education, Ltd.

To learn more about Cengage Learning Solutions, visit **www.cengage.com**.

Purchase any of our products at your local college store or at our preferred online store **www.cengagebrain.com**.

For product information and technology assistance, contact us at **Cengage Learning Customer & Sales Support, 1-800-354-9706**.

For permission to use material from this text or product, submit all requests online at **www.cengage.com/permissions** Further permissions questions can be emailed to **permissionrequest@cengage.com**.

Cover Image: ©Klemin Misic/Shutterstock

Printed in the United States of America
Print Number: 01   Print Year: 2014

Table of Contents

Introduction

Posttraumatic stress disorder (PTSD) became recognized as a diagnosis in 1980 in relation to veterans of war but is now related to other instances of trauma where one's life or that of another close person has been threatened with serious harm or lethality (Simpson, 2012, p. 13). In fact, the most common cause of PTSD is the sudden, unexpected loss of a loved one (Gabbard, 2000, p. 252). Interestingly, it appears that most people do not develop PTSD when faced with even the most horrifying trauma while others suffer from PTSD when faced with trauma relatively low in severity (Gabbard, 2000, p. 253). This is due to predisposing factors. An important consideration to keep in mind is that a person should not be diagnosed as suffering from PTSD merely because she or he has experienced a traumatic event. The Diagnostic and Statistical Manual of Mental Disorders (DSM-5) provides clear criteria of this disorder. The definition and criteria for PTSD will be discussed in the next section.

It is also possible for someone to develop PTSD following a physical or sexual assault on a loved one. This could be referred to as secondary PTSD or Secondary Trauma. The symptoms may be the same, thereby permitting a diagnosis of PTSD.

Prevalence

According to the 16th Annual National Center for PTSD Report (2012), 20-25% of those witnessing or experiencing a traumatic event will develop some stress-related symptoms. Approximately 8-10% will develop PTSD. In 80% of cases of PTSD, individuals also present with substance abuse, chronic pain, gastrointestinal issues, headaches and/or depression (Simpson, 2012, p. 13). The Anxiety and Depression Association of American (2013) state that 7.7 million Americans age 18 and older have PTSD and that 67% of people exposed to mass violence have been shown to develop PTSD, which is a higher rate than those exposed to natural disasters or other types of traumatic events.

Key Concepts

Acute Stress Disorder (ASD): The symptoms are the same as those for PTSD with a few differences. This diagnosis identifies people suffering from severe acute stress reactions in the period prior to when a diagnosis of PTSD can be made. The definition of ASD requires at least 9 out of 14 symptoms be present without regard to any particular cluster.

Affective: This refers to the emotional aspect of one's experiences and responses.

Alteration in arousal and reactivity: This is a symptom of PTSD in which the person shifts from total focus on the trauma through flashbacks, nightmares, and re-experiencing the trauma to becoming numb toward and dissociating from the event.

Anhedonia: This symptom of PTSD refers to the person's inability to feel pleasure in life. It is also a symptom of depression.

Avoidance: This symptom of PTSD refers to the person's tendency to stay away from any situation or cues that resemble the traumatic event.

Battered Women's Syndrome: Often, repeated episodes of abuse lead to this form of PTSD. The woman comes to believe that the situation is hopeless and that she can't do anything to fix it. She is afraid to leave because her husband may kill her or the children, for fear that she cannot survive on her own, or that family and friends will reject her if she leaves.

Child Abuse Accommodation Syndrome: This syndrome typically has five aspects to it. In the first phase, the child is abused. In the second phase, the perpetrator asks or demands that the child not tell anyone, hence securing secrecy from the child. In the third phase, the child accommodates the abuse and does not fight it or demand to be treated better. In the fourth phase, the abuse is somehow mentioned to someone, often by accident. This disclosure phase often precipitates a crisis in the child and parents. In the fifth and last phase, the child suppresses the disclosure by recanting his or her story of abuse. Often, the perpetrator tells the child to suppress the disclosure.

Cognitive: This refers to the thoughts, beliefs, and perceptions that a person holds about an event, themselves, or others.

Cognitive Processing Therapy: This type of therapy includes four primary components: education regarding a client's specific PTSD symptoms, increasing awareness of associated thoughts and feelings related to symptoms, skill-building to facilitate questioning or challenging the thoughts, and understanding changes in beliefs.

Critical incident and debriefing: This is a crisis intervention method that stabilizes, supports and normalizes people in an effort to strengthen their coping abilities, and hopefully, prevent long-term damage such as PTSD, substance abuse, depression, and family and relationship problems. It is not intended as treatment but is largely supportive and educational.

Delayed expression: This term is used when a full diagnosis is not met until at least six months after the trauma.

Depersonalization: The person experiences himself or herself as being an outside observer or detached from oneself (e.g., feeling as if "this is not happening to me" or in a dream).

Derealization: The person experiences life as not real, from a distance or with distortions (e.g. "things are not real").

Disaster mental health: Because of the extent of manmade and natural disasters, mental health professionals have developed special programs and training that focus on helping people and communities overcome the effects of traumas or critical incidents.

Dissociation: This symptom allows victims of trauma to compartmentalize the experience so that it is no longer accessible to consciousness; sometimes amnesia of the actual event occurs.

Dissociative Identity Disorder: This is a condition in which a person develops various alters or fragments of the self that are presented to the world. Amnesia often exists between alternate identities.

Dysphoria: This refers to a state of depression and feeling unhappy.

Eye movement desensitization and reprocessing (EMDR): This psychotherapy involves elements of exposure to traumatic stimuli via imaging and use of cognitive-behavioral methods.

Hypervigilance: This symptom of PTSD refers to a person being guarded and in an exaggerated state of preparedness to detect threats or a negative experience to happen.

Intrusion: These symptoms of PTSD deal with the person having unwelcome thoughts of the trauma and re-experiencing it.

Manmade disaster: These include accidents, like plane crashes, as well as those perpetrated with malicious intent—such as the Boston Marathon bombing in 2013 and the 9/11 terrorist attacks in 2001.

Military sexual trauma: This phrase was coined during the wars in Iraq and Afghanistan to refer to the many reported cases of sexual assault, rape, and harassment experienced, especially by women.

Natural disaster: Natural disasters include landslides, floods, fires, earthquakes, hurricanes, and other storm conditions that wreak havoc on humans.

Negative alteration in cognitions and mood: This symptom of PTSD refers to the tendency for the person to switch back and forth between thinking negatively about the trauma, often blaming themselves, and not being able to remember the trauma or aspects of the trauma.

Oscillation: This term refers to the back and forth, alternating, and switching moods, thoughts, and focus that people with PTSD often experience.

Prolonged Exposure Therapy (PET): This approach involves having survivors repeatedly re-experience their traumatic event. It includes both imaginary exposure and in vivo exposure to safe situations that have been avoided because they elicit traumatic reminders.

Rape Trauma Syndrome (RTS): The process in RTS is similar to ASD, then PTSD. In the first stage, the woman experiences the overwhelming shock of the assault and shows signs of all of the symptoms of ASD. After about one month, without intervention, the woman will reorganize and use defense mechanisms such as repression, dissociation, denial, minimization, and somatization to ward off the debilitating effects of the rape. She then enters into the PTSD stage. She may remain functioning at this lower level the rest of her life or may seek treatment at some point until she can learn to integrate the trauma, the final stage of RTS.

Regression: This term refers to the tendency for a person to return to earlier modes of coping and behaving during times of stress.

Secondary Trauma Syndrome/Compassion Fatigue: People who regularly work with individuals in crisis situations may be prone to develop symptoms of PTSD.

Stress inoculation training: The three phases of the training include the initial establishment of trust and a collaborative relationship between the client and clinician, encouraging the client to view symptoms as problems to be addressed and solved—through which the client is taught to analyze a problem into small manageable parts—and developing long-term coping skills.

Stressor: This refers to a trauma that occurs that often leads to PTSD. When the event has a life threatening aspect to it, PTSD may occur after the event.

Trauma and Stressor-related Disorders: The required criteria of exposure to trauma links the conditions included in this classification.

Definition of PTSD and Diagnostic Criteria

PTSD is a broad category that applies to people who have been severely traumatized at one or more times in their lives and are not functioning effectively because they have not integrated the trauma. The Diagnostic and Statistical Manual of Mental Disorders (DSM-5) (American Psychiatric Association, 2013), provides the criteria for an individual to warrant this diagnosis. The latest DSM revision now includes a preschool subtype for children six years and younger. The DSM-5 also added a new dissociative subtype for adults, but still retained the delayed expression subtype. The criteria for adults and those older than six are described below. Symptoms of PTSD in children six and younger will be discussed later. In general, PTSD criteria include exposure to a traumatic event and symptoms related to intrusion, avoidance, negative alterations in cognitions and mood, and alterations in arousal and reactivity.

Additionally, duration of the symptoms, functioning level and issues of substance or co-occurring medical condition factor into a PTSD diagnosis. Below are the eight criteria according to the DSM-5:

A. **Stressor:** A person must have been exposed to death, threatened by death, actual or threatened serious injury, or actual or threatened sexual violence either by:

   1) direct exposure,

   2) witnessing in person, and/or

   3) indirectly by learning that a close relative or friend was exposed to trauma as long as the actual or threatened death involved was violent or accidental.

B. **Intrusion symptoms:** The traumatic event must be persistently re-experienced in at least one of the following ways:

1) recurrent, involuntary and intrusive memories (children older than 6 may express this in repetitive play,

2) traumatic nightmares (children may have frightening dreams without content related to the trauma),

3) dissociative reactions (e.g. flashbacks) which may occur on a continuum from brief episodes to complete loss of consciousness (children may reenact the event in play),

4) intense or prolonged distress after exposure to traumatic reminders, and/or

5) marked physiologic reactivity after exposure to trauma-related stimuli.

C. **Avoidance:** The person experiences at least one persistent effortful avoidance of distressing trauma-related stimuli after the event, such as:

1) trauma-related thoughts or feelings and/or

2) trauma-related external reminders (e.g. people, places, conversations, activities, objects, or situations).

D. **Negative alterations in cognitions and mood**: The person experiences at least two of the following symptoms that are indicative of negative alterations in cognitions and mood that began or worsened after the traumatic event:

1) inability to recall key features of the traumatic event (usually dissociative amnesia, not due to head injury, alcohol, or drugs),

2) persistent (and often distorted) negative beliefs and expectations about oneself or the world (e.g., "I am bad." "the world is completely dangerous."),

3) persistent distorted blame of self or others for causing the traumatic event or for resulting consequences,

4) persistent negative trauma-related emotions (e.g., fear, horror, anger, guilt, or shame),

5) markedly diminished interest in (pre-traumatic) significant activities,

6) feeling alienated from others (e.g., detachment or estrangement), and/or

7) constricted affect, which is the persistent inability to experience positive emotions.

E. **Alterations in arousal and reactivity:** The person experiences at least two of the following trauma-related alterations in arousal and reactivity that began or worsened after the traumatic event:

1) irritable or aggressive behavior,

2) self-destructive or reckless behavior,

3) hypervigilance,

4) exaggerated startle response,

5) problems concentrating, and/or

6) sleep disturbance

F. **Duration:** The symptoms in the above criteria must have existed for more than one month.

G. **Functional significance:** The person experiences significant symptom-related distress or functional impairment socially, occupationally, academically, behaviorally, and so on.

H. **Exclusion:** The disturbance is not due to medication, substance use, or other illness.

Additionally, the person experiences high levels of one of the following dissociative symptoms:

1. **Depersonalization:** The person experiences him or herself as being an outside observer of or detached from oneself (e.g., feeling as if "this is not happening to me" or one were in a dream).

2. **Derealization:** The person experiences life as not real, from a distance or with distortions (e.g. "things are not real").

Lastly, the diagnosing clinician must specify if the PTSD is with **delayed expression** where a full diagnosis is not met until at least six months after the trauma.

Revisions

The release of the DSM-5 in May 2013 suggests that the information above is the most current. Although the criteria are similar to those listed in DSM-IV, there are some major revisions to the PTSD diagnosis based on scientific research and clinical experiences. Below are the major revisions to the PTSD diagnosis from DSM-IV to DSM-5. (Incidentally, it may be worth noting that instead of using Roman numerals to indicate the 5th edition, the APA is now using Arabic numerals).

1. Classification: PTSD and ASD (to be discussed further later) both moved from the class of anxiety disorders into a new class, **trauma and stressor-related disorders**. This change was based on the clinical recognition of variable expressions of distress as a result of traumatic experience. The required criteria of exposure to trauma links the conditions included in this classification. In addition to the anxiety or fear-based symptoms, individuals suffering from PTSD and ASD typically experience anxiety symptoms such as **anhedonia** and **dysphoria,** anger and aggression, **dissociation,** or some combination of these (U.S. Department of Veterans Affairs, 2013).

2. Diagnostic criteria: Overall, the symptoms of both of these trauma and stressor-related disorders have remained the same in DSM-5 compared to DSM-IV. Some revisions are presented below:

   a. In DSM-IV there were only three clusters of symptoms, while in DSM-5 there are four clusters: intrusion, avoidance, negative alterations in cognitions and mood, and alterations in arousal and reactivity. The DSM-IV criterion C, avoidance and numbing, was separated into two of the DSM-5 Criteria C (avoidance) and D (negative alterations in cognitions and mood).

   b. Three new symptoms were added: In Criteria D (negative alterations in cognitions and mood): 1.) persistent and distorted blame of self or others, and 2.) persistent negative emotional state. In Criteria E (alterations in arousal and reactivity) 3.) reckless or destructive behavior.

3. Criterion A2 (requiring fear, helplessness, or horror happen right after the trauma) was not included in DSM-5.

4. A clinical subtype "with dissociative symptoms" was added for those who meet the criteria for PTSD and experience additional depersonalization and derealization symptoms.

5. Separate diagnostic criteria are included in DSM-5 for children ages 6 years or younger (preschool subtype).

6. Criterion A1 in DSM-5 narrowed qualifying traumatic events such that the unexpected death of family or a close friend due to natural causes is no longer included.

Acute Stress Disorder (ASD)

Acute Stress Disorder is another syndrome in the classification of trauma and stress-related disorders. The symptoms of this are the same as those for PTSD with a few differences. ASD was initially introduced in DSM-IV for two reasons: to describe severe acute stress reactions that occur in the initial month after a traumatic event that could not be described as PTSD (which requires that more than a month has passed since the event), and to identify acutely traumatized people who will subsequently develop PTSD as opposed to experiencing a transient stress reaction (Spiegel et al., 1996). ASD was differentiated from PTSD by a strong emphasis on acute dissociation. One needed to have at least three of the following symptoms of dissociation to be diagnosed with ASD: emotional numbing, derealization, depersonalization, reduced awareness of surroundings, or dissociative amnesia. While overall the ASD diagnosis is sensitive in predicting PTSD; that is, the majority of people with a diagnosis of ASD do subsequently develop PTSD (Bryant, 2013), most people who eventually experience PTSD do not initially display ASD. Why is this the case? It may have been the overemphasis on dissociative symptoms required in the DSM-IV for diagnosing ASD. Many people at risk for PTSD do not display acute dissociative responses (Bryant, et al., 2008).

As a result of accumulating evidence that ASD does not accurately predict long-term PTSD, the DSM-5 has modified the goals and criteria for ASD. This diagnosis no longer attempts to predict chronic PTSD but identifies people suffering from severe acute stress reactions in the period prior to when a diagnosis of PTSD can be made. The new definition of ASD now requires at least 9 out of 14 symptoms without regard to any particular cluster. For a diagnosis of ASD, individuals can experience a range of traumatic stress responses that may or may not include dissociative symptoms (Bryant, et al., 2011). However, the diagnosis of

9

ASD still requires some form of re-experiencing and/or avoidance. Overall, ASD and PTSD generally remain the same clinically with time following trauma being the most important difference.

Psychodynamic Theory of PTSD

M. J. Horowitz (1976) studied the impact of trauma on personality and observed that trauma victims alternate between denying the event and compulsively repeating it through flashbacks or nightmares. He hypothesized that this was the mind's attempt to process and organize overwhelming stimuli. He further proposes that most people do not develop PTSD even when faced with horrifying trauma, so there must be certain predisposing factors such as genetic makeup, childhood trauma, personality characteristics, compromised support system, and perceptions where locus of control is external rather than internal.

G. O. Gabbard (2000, p. 253) suggests that although dissociative defenses may be activated to keep intense, painful affects out of awareness, the salience of traumatic memories causes them to be maintained at a high state of cognitive activation. He presents the idea that **cognitive** and **affective** factors may work at cross-purposes and lead to the **oscillation** between memory intrusion and memory failure common in individuals suffering from PTSD. Sigmund Freud postulated the repetition compulsion as the source of intrusive traumatic memories in his original psychoanalytic theory. However, more current psychodynamic theory concludes that unresolved traumatic memories remain cognitively activated precisely because they are affectively inhibited by defense mechanisms such as dissociation. Gabbard further suggests that the unconscious monitoring system that keeps traumatic memories at bay because of their associations with painful affective states also assumes that they cannot be worked through.

Modern psychodynamic views of PTSD have been influenced by the work of Henry Krystal (1988). In his view, psychic trauma in childhood results in an arrest of affective development, whereas trauma in adulthood leads to a **regression** in affective development. The end result of both situations is that survivors of trauma cannot use affects as signals because powerful emotion is viewed as a threat that the original trauma will return. They can no longer soothe themselves in order to sleep or relax and stay calm.

Defense mechanisms, another psychodynamic concept related to PTSD, are used to overcome the feeling of being a victim. The victim often projects their own rage onto others and sustains a hypervigilant stance in an effort to protect themselves from the aggression they perceive in those around them. Guilt may also be used as a defense, like when a rape victim assumes responsibility for the rape thereby masking the disturbing thought that she was completely helpless in a universe where violence is random.

Physiology of PTSD

Sensory input, memory formation, and stress response mechanisms have been affected in patients with PTSD. The regions of the brain involved in memory processing likely the cause of these changes in PTSD include the limbic system and the frontal cortex. The heightened stress response is likely to involve the limbic system (Fighting PTSD, 2013). The limbic system is sometimes referred to as the "emotional brain" and is located deep within the cerebrum. It is composed of the amygdala, the hippocampus, and the hypothalamus—which are involved in the expression of emotions and motivation, particularly those related to survival. Fear, anger and the "fight or flight" response as well as feelings of pleasure that reward behaviors related to species survival are in this system. The limbic system has functions related to memory storage and retrieval, particularly when the memories relate to events that evoke strong emotional responses.

The amygdala seems to be genetically different and "wired" for a higher level of fear in some people, such as those with PTSD. MRI studies have shown marked changes in the hippocampus in the brain of those with PTSD that is thought to be caused by increased exposure to cortisol (the stress hormone). This part of the limbic system is responsible for transferring information into autobiographical and fact memory. The fact that it may be changed in those with PTSD explains memory failure often seen in PTSD.

Fishman (2013) discusses the effects of these changes in the brain and limbic system on a person with PTSD. Since PTSD leads to prolonged stress both physiologically and psychologically, it comes as no surprise that being in a constant state of arousal is hard on the cardiovascular system. Stress increases heart rate and blood pressure. PTSD victims, specifically war veterans, have an increased risk of dying from coronary heart disease. Additionally, feelings of depression and constant anxiety in those with PTSD may lead them to run to illegal drugs or smoking to alleviate symptoms. In fact, they tend to smoke more than non-PTSD sufferers. PTSD also seems to have implications for the immune system in that they have more inflammation within the body and a higher white blood cell count that can lead to blood disorders or serious infections. When the body is in a constant state of fight or flight, the immune system is overactive. They may also have a higher risk of cancer and autoimmune disease as well as early mortality.

Potential Traumas that Often Lead to PTSD

One of the unique aspects of a PTSD diagnosis is the importance placed upon the causal agent, the traumatic stressor. One cannot make a PTSD diagnosis unless this stressor criterion has been met. Because not everyone develops PTSD even when exposed to the same stressor, it has been hypothesized that trauma may be filtered through cognitive processes before it is appraised as an extreme threat and there are individual differences in this appraisal process. People have different trauma thresholds (Yarvis, 2013, p. 83). As suggested earlier, sudden loss of a loved one may cause PTSD. When this is the stressor, the PTSD is complicated by grief. Not only does the person need to deal with the PTSD, the sufferer must also work through the stages of mourning. It is not surprising that a large number of PTSD sufferers also express feeling depressed. Many traumas include a loss of some type whether it be loss of material possessions, loss of a loved one, loss of safety, loss of a limb, and so on. In addition to sudden, unexpected death of a loved one, PTSD may follow a number of traumatic events. For example, as of 2011, in the military, the PTSD diagnosis no longer requires a specific experience of a specific event with verifiable time and date. The ongoing exposure to war itself can justify the diagnosis. Other experiences that make someone vulnerable to PTSD may include but are not limited to : early childhood trauma, fatal car accident, natural disasters involving traumatic loss, physical or sexual assault on self or loved ones, family violence, domestic violence and random social violence (Simpson, 2012), such as mass gun shootings or terrorist attacks. Even having one's home burglarized, being robbed at gunpoint, being kidnapped or being a parent of a child who is abducted, witnessing or being part of a gruesome car accident may make someone vulnerable to PTSD (Kanel, 2015). Remember, when the individual seeks help within a month after a traumatic event and demonstrates symptoms of PTSD, s/he should be given the ASD diagnosis. When they wait more than a month for treatment and have been experiencing the symptoms of PTSD, then that diagnosis is warranted.

Following is a discussion of a variety of traumatic events that often lead to PTSD. Various prevalence rates, facts, and phenomenological experiences are also presented.

Military Combat: It is fair to suggest that the average person associates PTSD with combat veterans. Indeed, those serving in the military frequently experience symptoms of ASD while serving and continue with those symptoms upon return to civilian life; hence manifesting symptoms of PTSD. The term PTSD was first coined in the 1980 DSM III as a way to provide a diagnosis for the many Vietnam veterans who suffered from PTSD for years following that war. This syndrome had been referred to as "shell shock" when discussing the signs of trauma exhibited by World War II veterans (Kanel, 2015). The most recent wars in Iraq and Afghanistan have been said to be an incubator for PTSD; therefore understanding the particular issues facing the hundreds of thousands of military personnel returning due to the recent and continuing drawdowns makes it essential to provide mental health providers about the special needs and best treatment practices for this population. An entire chapter is devoted to these issues later in these series of chapters.

Another unique aspect to these current wars is the fact that woman have served in vast numbers, especially in comparison to other wars. This has led to a surge in reported cases of sexual assaults. The term **Military Sexual Trauma (MST)** has been coined to refer to these situations. Woman suffering from MST are more likely to develop PTSD than those who did not. While the issue of rape/sexual assault will be discussed below, and most of that information is relevant to MST, there are other complicating factors related to the military culture that make MST unique from other sexual assaults. MST will be addressed in detail in the chapter on veteran's issues.

Personal Victimization: We turn now to situations in which an individual is threatened to be assaulted or is actually assaulted physically, sexually, or both by another. These situations are complicated as the perpetrator is frequently someone that the victim knows, such as a relative or acquaintance. Not only does the survivor of these assaults have to deal with thoughts of being powerless and helpless, but they must often deal with conflicting feelings of rage and love toward a loved one. Additionally, because these assaults are a crime, the victim must make decisions about how to proceed legally and deal with the criminal justice system and at times the child protective system. Whether or not to report the assault to the authorities further complicates the situation, especially when the victim is suffering from PTSD. While in a state of dissociation and hypervigilance, the victim is not in the best state of mind to navigate these many complexities and often requires the assistance of professionals.

Each of these types of victimizations has their own particular form of PTSD. Many rape survivors often develop **Rape Trauma Syndrome**; which follows the path from Acute Stress Disorder (ASD) to PTSD. Women who live in an ongoing abusive relationship with a husband, boyfriend, or other type of mate, often develop Battered Women's Syndrome. When someone is first battered, ASD may develop, but after many years of experiencing the assaults, the individual copes by numbing and dissociating from the abuse. In many cases they develop PTSD with symptoms of depression, feelings of helplessness, and learning to live to survive rather than escape. This is when **Battered Women's Syndrome** exists; in essence a form of PTSD. Lastly, children who are physically or sexually abuse also present with their own unique form of PTSD, sometimes referred to as **Child Abuse Accommodation Syndrome.** They learn to numb themselves to the abuse, dissociate from it, and maintain secrecy. When children are subjected to chronic sexual, physical, and emotional abuse by those they live with for many years, the PTSD may develop into a serious condition, **Dissociative Identity Disorder (DID)** in which they develop various alters/fragments of the self that are presented to the world. This differs from PTSD in that person suffers from amnesia regularly and is unaware of the other alters for the most part. DID is rare and occurs when the abuse is ongoing by loved ones with no one available to provide any support to the child, because it is the parents that are the perpetrators.

> 1. Rape/Sexual Assault: Most sexual-assault victims are females, though men can also be victims of sexual assault, especially in prison. This section deals only with adult victims of sexual assault. Sexual assault occurs when one person forces any sexual behavior on another. This can include many types of forced physical contact, including rape (forced vaginal or anal penetration), forced oral copulation, and other sexual acts that one person is forcing on another.
>
> *Prevalence:* According to worldwide estimates, at least one in three women has been beaten, coerced into sex, or otherwise abused during her lifetime (Heise, Ellsberg, & Gottemoeller, 1999).

According to the U.S. Bureau of Justice (2013):

- From 1995 to 2010, the estimated annual rate of female rape or sexual assault victimizations declined 58% from 5.0 victimizations per 1,000 females age 12 or older to 2.1 per 1,000.

- Females 34 years or younger living in lower income households in rural areas had the highest rates of sexual violence from 2005–2010.

- From 2005 to 2010, the offender was armed with a gun, knife, or other weapon in 11% of rape cases.

- From 2005 to 2010, 78% of sexual violence involved an offender who was a family member, intimate partner, friend, or acquaintance.

- 57% of rapes happen on dates.

- 84% of rape victims tried unsuccessfully to reason with the man t raped her.

- 55% of gang rapes on college campuses are committed by fraternities, 40% by sports teams and 5% by others.

- In the 1980s, 5% of rape survivors went to the police.

- In the past 10 years, 30% of rape survivors report it to the police.

- Of those who report it, 5% of the time a man who rapes ends up in prison, 95% of the time he does not.

- 42% of rape survivors had sex again with the rapist.

- 30% of rape survivors contemplate suicide after the rape.

- 82% of rape survivors say the rape permanently changed them.

- The adult pregnancy rate associated with rape is 4.7%.

- 89,000 rape cases are reported annually.

- 16% of women experienced an attempted or completed rape.

- 3% of men experienced an attempted or completed rape.

- There is a 60% decline in rapes since 1993.

While some may still blame the victim for being raped, claiming that she is promiscuous, or a scorned lover, or that she was provocative, most social scientists do not hold these views. Instead, the rape victim is viewed as not having anything to do with being raped. She is simply a victim of a rapist who has needs to control and humiliate. Her only role is being female, weak physically, and perhaps too trusting. Some propose that a woman who is raped may not have the psychological resources to protect herself. She may be in shock once attacked and not be able to yell or fight. This may be a survival mechanism that could save her life. Date rape is the most common type of rape. A woman may simply not know she is being raped. Some women believe that if they agree to talk with a man, kiss a man, get close physically with a man, or even engage in heavy petting, they are required to "go all the way." They do not know that they have the right to say "no" at any time (Kanel, 2015). Lack of knowledge, then, is another factor that may play a part in sexual assault. The traumatic aspect of date rape is that the woman just was not expecting things to get out of hand. It is a shock to her psychological system. This shock is an aspect of the physiology of PTSD discussed above.

Perceiving oneself as having been helpless and powerless are the common cognitions in rape survivors associated with PTSD, or as mentioned above, Rape Trauma Syndrome (RTS). The process in RTS is similar to ASD, then PTSD. In the first stage, the woman experiences the overwhelming shock of the assault and shows signs of all of the symptoms of ASD. After about one month, without intervention, the woman will reorganize and use defense mechanisms such as repression, dissociation, denial, minimization, and somatization to ward of the debilitating effects of the rape. She then enters into the PTSD stage. She may remain functioning at this lower level the rest of her life or may seek treatment at some point until she can learn to integrate the trauma, the final stage of RTS.

2. Interpersonal Partner Abuse: This section focuses on females who are abused by male partners. While men do live in abusive relationships with women, most would agree that women are at far greater risk of severe if not fatal injury from partner abuse than men are. This is due in part to a man's physical size and strength, which make him less physically intimidated by a woman. However, men may be subject to emotional abuse by women at the same rate as women are by men. So while this section focuses on women being abused by men, keep in mind that domestic abuse can occur in situations where two men are living together, two women are living together, and to men who are living with an abusive woman. The bottom line is that when someone perceives themselves to be

threatened or experiences some form of physical assault, they are vulnerable to developing PTSD.

Prevalence: Some statistical information might give the reader a general idea of how prevalent domestic violence is in the United States. Safe Horizon (2013) offers some facts about domestic violence:

- One in four women will experience domestic violence in her lifetime.
- Women are more likely than men to be killed by an intimate partner.
- Women ages 20–24 are at greatest risk of becoming victims of domestic violence.
- Every year, one in three women who is a victim of homicide is murdered by her current or former partner.
- Every year, more than 3 million children witness domestic violence in their homes.
- Children who live in homes where there is domestic violence also suffer high rates of abuse or neglect (30–60%).
- More than 60% of domestic violence incidents happen at home.
- Domestic violence is the 3rd leading cause of homelessness.
- Domestic violence costs more than $37 billion a year in law enforcement involvement, legal work, medical and mental health treatment and lost productivity at companies.
- Most domestic violence incidents are never reported!

Battered-women's syndrome: Walker (1984) proposed that women stay in battering relationships because they suffer from battered-women's syndrome, which results from repeated episodes of abuse. The woman comes to believe that the situation is hopeless and that she can't do anything to fix it. She is afraid to leave because her husband may kill her or the children, for fear that she cannot survive on her own or that family and friends will reject her if she leaves. She may also believe that she loves her husband and that the children need their father. Many of these beliefs are irrational and can be altered through cognitive therapy. These feelings of helplessness, hopelessness, and worthlessness cause women to live in a chronic state of emptiness and shock, focusing only on survival rather than escape. This lifestyle is similar to that of a prisoner of war. Both tend to blame themselves and seek their captor's approval without thought of escape. Battered women's syndrome looks much like PTSD. Sometimes when a woman experiences violence against her, she will show symptoms of ASD as well. Over time, if she remains in the relationship, she survives by dissociation, repression, and other defenses that are part of PTSD. Even when she escapes the relationship, she will manifest symptoms of PTSD.

3. Child Abuse: If child abuse is not detected and brought to the attention of mental health workers, the abused individual often develops symptoms of PTSD following the abuse, which often continue into adulthood. The trauma of being abused often affects a person's functioning in work and personal relationships. Often, adults who were sexually abused as children (or adults molested as children (AMACS)) may unwittingly repeat the abuse with their own children or perpetuate abuse on themselves. Suicide and substance abuse are commonly associated with these individuals as well. As children, denying the abuse helped in their daily survival, but as adults, denial often works against their surviving daily stress.

Many children who are repeatedly abused develop Child Abuse Accommodation Syndrome as described earlier. In order to not feel the emotional torment of being abused, neglected, and sexually abused, the child protects himself or herself by accepting the abuse and not fighting it. Abuse can continue for many years before it gets reported. Sometimes it is never reported, and victims die with the secret of having been a victim of abuse. When it does get reported, it is often by accident. The family is not ready psychologically to handle the disclosure and everyone goes into a crisis state. All family members use defenses: dissociation, repressions, denial, minimization, and externalization to maintain a stable family. However, it is the child that develops this type of PTSD, the primary symptoms being dissociation, repression, and numbing. They are also often very angry as they develop into adults and may repeat the abuse with their own children if the PTSD goes untreated.

Child Abuse Accommodation Syndrome: In order to emotionally and psychological survive the trauma of chronic sexual/physical abuse or neglect, many children accommodate the abuse and numb themselves to their feelings. They live in a dissociated state, detached from emotional pain. This syndrome typically has five aspects to it. In the first phase, the child is abused. In the second phase, the perpetrator asks or demands that the child not tell anyone, hence securing secrecy from the child. In the third phase, the child accommodates the abuse and does not fight it or demand to be treated better. In the fourth phase, the abuse is somehow mentioned to someone, often by accident. This disclosure phase often precipitates a crisis in the child and parents. In the fifth and last phase, the child suppresses the disclosure by recanting his/her story of abuse. Often, the perpetrator tells the child to suppress the disclosure.

In general, children manifest symptoms of PTSD differently than adults; that is why the DSM-5 added a section on children in its discussion on PTSD. Some of the symptoms common in young children after a trauma or abuse include:

- Returning to earlier behaviors, such as thumbsucking or bedwetting
- Clinging to parents
- Being reluctant to go to bed
- Having nightmares
- Having fantasies that the trauma never happened
- Ccrying and screaming
- Withdrawing and becoming immobile
- Refusing to attend school
- Having problems at school and being unable to concentrate (American Red Cross, 2001)

Additionally, because abused children are usually traumatized by parents, they are prone to feelings of shame—a result of disattunement with caretakers. Prolonged and repeated shame-states result in a physiological dysregulation that negatively impacts the development of networks of affective regulation and attachment circuitry. Shame leads to feeling sociallly excluded, which is painful and stimulates the same areas of our brains that become active when we experience physical pain (Cozolino, 2006, as cited in Walker, 2011, p. 452).

Living Through a Natural Disaster: Natural disasters include landslides, floods, fires, earthquakes, hurricanes, and other storm conditions that wreak havoc on humans. A recent example is devastating Hurricane Sandy, which caused billions of dollars worth of damage, primarily in the New Jersey area. As a result of the mismanagement of Hurricane Katrina of 2005, which nearly destroyed the city of New Orleans and caused billions of dollars worth of damage in several states bordering the Gulf of Mexico, the federal government seemed to provide services more rapidly and effectively to the victims of Sandy. While survivors of Sandy no doubt suffered, and some probably are suffering from PTSD, the flooding of a large area of New Orleans left thousands of people homeless and without food, water, and electricity for several days, until rescue workers arrived to help evacuate those stranded. The potential for PTSD may have been increased due to living days without services and perceived lack of help from the govenrment. The perception that the federal administration was prepared to offer resources was vital in helping the Sandy victims deal with that disaster emotionally. This contrasts with the vitcims of Katrina believing that the federal govenmenr was not offering services and didn't seem to care (Kanel, 2015, p. 157-158).

Natural disasters have occurred throughout history and will no doubt continue. Many people have been traumatized by the pwerful destruction of earthquakes, blizzards, storms, and floods. These types of disasters make people feel helpless and they may even become angry with God.

When a disaster hits, communities tend to go through certain phases to overcome the psychological and physical consequences of the disaster. The Mental Health Center of North Iowa, Inc. (retrieved 6/8/2005) provides information about these phases. The first stage is the heroic phase. This usually occurs during and immediately after the disaster. Emotions are strong and direct. People find themselves being called upon for and responding to demands for heroic action to save their own and others' lives and property. Altruism is prominent, and people expend much energy in helping others to survive and recover. People have a lot of energy and motivation to help. Everyone pitches in to help people that they might not ordinarily have assisted. The second stage is the honeymoon phase, which lasts from one week to six months after the disaster. There is a strong sense of having shared with others a dangerous, catastrophic experience and having lived through it. Survivors clean out mud and debris from their homes and yards, anticipating that a considerable amount of help will soon be given them to solve their problems. Community groups that are set up to meet specific needs caused by the disaster are important resources during this period. The third stage is the disillusionment phase. When the "honeymoon high" wears off, people realize that life isn't a "bowl of cherries." They realize that people have returned to their normal states of greed, jealousy, and selfishness. The "utopia" they had envisioned doesn't materialize. Strong feelings of disappointment, anger, resentment, and bitterness may arise if promised aid is delayed or never arrives. Outside agencies may leave the affected region, and some community groups may weaken or may not adapt to the changing situation. There is a gradual loss of the feelings of "shared community" as survivors concentrate on rebuilding their lives and solving their own individual problems. The final stage is the reconstruction phase, in which survivors realize that they will need to rebuild their homes, businesses, and lives largely by themselves, and gradually assume the responsibility for doing so. This phase might last for several years following the disaster. Community support groups are essential during this phase as well. Of course, survivors of natural disasters may develop ASD within the first month after the disaster and then some develop PTSD after the first month. Clinicals must assess the phase of community support when working with PTSD sufferers following both natural and manmade disasters.

Manmade Disasters: Crisis work began when a manmade disaster, the Coconut Grove Nightclub fire, occurred in 1942 (Kanel, 2015). Approximately 500 people died in that fire, leaving survivors in shock and grief. Gerald Caplan and Eric Lindemann created the Wellesley project in response to that disaster as a place to study reactions to traumas and how to help people work through them. The term PTSD had not yet been utilized. Caplan coined the term "preventive psychiatry" when talking about crisis management. Based on what we now understand about unexpected loss of loved ones being a high risk indicator for developing PTSD, it is highly probably that many of the survivors of that nightclub fire did suffer from ASD and PTSD. Caplan and Lindemann had some success in treating thsese survivors in much the same way current trauma workers implement critical incident and debriefing for survivors of natural and man-made disasters. Many disasters of this magnitude or worse have occurred since the fire. Sometimes they are accidental, as when a plane crashes; others are perpetrated on purpose and with malicious intent.

1. World Trade Center and Pentagon Attacks: One such manmade disaster was the terrorist-hijacked airplane crashes into the New York World Trade Center and the U.S. Pentagon on September 11, 2001. These traumas lead to the death of over 5,000 people, the highest disaster-related death toll in U.S. history. Most of us can still remember how the entire country proceeded through the different phases discussed above. The pictures are etched in our minds of men and women working day and night to remove debris from

the areas affected by the attacks. This behavior helped to increase feelings of power in all of us. At least something could be done. Unfortunately, this tragedy did not end with the plane crashes but continued with the introduction by terrorists of the anthrax virus into the U.S. Postal System. In 2005, terrorists left bombs in backpacks in the London transit system, reminding us that the threat continues (Kanel, 2015, p. 160).

2. Boston Bombing in 2013: A more recent manmade disaster was the Boston Marathon terrorist bombing that occurred in 2013. What a shock to have a wonderful afternoon ruined by two men who decided they had a right to kill and maim people due to religious and political motivations. This bombing was the first that took place since 9/11, and many were affected by it, perhaps some had a resurgence of their own PTSD due to its resemblance to the attacks on the World Trade Center (Kanel, 2015, p. 159).

3. Gun Violence and Shootings: Unfortunately, mass gun shootings have become all too common in our society. Each time we hear about one of these shootings, we all feel just a little less safe. Any of us are susceptible to developing PTSD or ASD after a shooting because they are often random. Who could have been prepared for the senseless killings of 20 children and 6 adults at Sandy Hook Elementary School in Newtown, Connecticut which took place in 2012? How do students and faculty at Virginia Tech University overcome feelings of threat after 32 people were murdered in a mass shooting in 2007? Hypervigilance, a PTSD symptom, makes sense for survivors of these situations. It is the mind's way of being prepared to survive if needed.

4. Oklahoma City Federal Building Bombing: The bombing of the Oklahoma City federal building in April 1995 is yet another example of a monumental disaster, in which more than 200 people, including preschool children, were killed and many others injured.

When disasters happen, they affect not only those directly involved but others who suddenly feel that their security is threatened. Communities throughout the United States responded to the recent traumatic events by providing much needed support.

Examples of community support included relief funds for families of the victims, generous donations to the Red Cross, and crisis response units established in a variety of locales such as elementary schools and even public parks. The crisis intervention was aimed at helping children and adults deal with beliefs that the community is no longer a safe place. Shock that something like this could happen to "me and my family" was a common response by manyvictims. Crisis workers needed to help people think differently about the situation, showing the secondary victims through education and empowerment statements that they could cope with this situation. Providing this help quickly may help overcome ASD before it turns into full-blown PTSD.

However, some people must put their feelings and normal human reactions aside following an emergency. This state of denial allows individuals to act in order to survive. If this initial shock and denial did not exist, people would be so overwhelmed with feelings that they could not function at all. After the emergency is stabilized, those involved can come to terms at an appropriate pace with what has happened. This process is referred to as a delayed PTSD.

The tendency is for individuals who have been traumatized to seek resolution at some point in some way. This resolution takes a variety of forms and may occur at conscious as well as unconscious levels. For example, nightmares that replay the event are common in PTSD. It is as if the unconscious mind is trying to help the person bring closure to the trauma by creating stress at night so the person will be motivated to deal with the trauma in a wakeful, conscious state.

Once individuals have allowed the trauma to surface, floods of feelings are aroused. Professional help is then needed to channel those feelings into productive avenues for growth. As with all crisis situations, people need to see that some new meaning can be ascribed to even the most devastating trauma. Victor Frankl's work on logotherapy (meaning therapy) is a good example; it shows how he used his trauma as a Nazi concentration camp survivor to create growth in himself as a person. Despite the catastrophic nature of his experience, he found a way to see meaning in it. This ability no doubt helped him survive psychologically.

If people do not receive help after a trauma, the posttraumatic symptoms get worse over time, and the individuals learn to adjust to life in a less functional way. Such people will have less psychic energy available for dealing with daily stresses, because they are using their energy to continue to deny the feelings associated with the trauma. These people will most likely have difficulty in interpersonal relationships, which require feelings if they are to be at all satisfying (Kanel, 2015, p. 163).

Critical Incident and Debriefing: Because of the extent of manmade and natural disasters, mental health professionals have developed special programs and training that focus on helping people and communities overcome the effects of traumas or critical incidents. All of the traumas discussed so far in this chapter are examples of critical incidents. Some mental health professionals refer to this process as trauma response or disaster mental health (Ladrech, 2004). Special training programs are available for workers wanting to help victims of disasters through the Red Cross and other responding organizations such as the International Medical Corps. Disaster mental health is a crisis intervention method that "stabilizes, supports and normalizes people in an effort to strengthen their coping abilities, and hopefully, prevent long-term damage such as PTSD, substance abuse, depression, and family and relationship problems. It is not meant to be treatment." (Ladrech, 2004, p. 21).

Best Clinical Practices in Treating PTSD

It has been found that cognitive-behavioral therapy leads to the most effective outcomes for people suffering from PTSD. Cognitive behavioral treatments typically include a number of components inlcuding psychoeducation, anxiety management, exposure, and cognitive restructuring. The Department of Veterans Affairs (DVA, 2012) agrees that cognitive behavioral treatments are the most effective. The best clinical practices in treating PTSD put forth by the DVA include Cognitive Processing Therapy, Prolonged Exposure Therapy, Eye Movement Desensitization Reprocessing, and Stress Reduction Inoculation Therapy. Each will be discussed below:

Cognitive Processing Therapy (CPT) is one of the most well researched cognitive approaches. The primary focus is on challenging and modifying maladaptive beliefs related to the trauma. This type of therapy includes four primary components: education regarding a client's specific PTSD symptoms, increasing awareness of associated thoughts and feelings related to symptoms, skill-building to facilitate questioning or challenging the thoughts, and understanding changes in beliefs. By working through these steps, the clinician and client explore how trauma impacted the person and how perspective may be changed to enhance healthy daily functioning (Simpson, 2013, p. 14). Ehlers & Clark (2000) have developed a cognitive therapy for PTSD that involved three goals: modifying excessively negative appraisals, correcting autobiographical memory disturbances, and removing problematic behavioral and cognitive strategies. Their therapy includes performing actions that are incompatible with the memory or engaging in behavioral experiments. Cognitive restructuring helps people make sense of the bad memories. Sometimes people remember the event differently than how it happened. They may feel guilt or shame about what is not their fault. The therapist helps people with PTSD look at what happened in a realistic way (Anxiety and Depression Association of America (ADAA), 2013).

Prolonged Exposure Therapy (PE): Exposure and cognitive restructuring are thought to be the most effective components of cognitive behavioral therapy (Hamblen, Schnurr, Rosenberg, & Eftekhari, 2013). These researchers assert that the greatest number of studies has been conducted on exposure-based treatments, which involve having survivors repeatedly re-experience their traumatic event. It includes both imaginal exposure and in vivo exposure to safe situations that have been avoided because they elicit traumatic reminders. As the name implies, this approach relies on repeated exposure to thoughts, feelings, and situations associated with the trauma, which the client may be avoiding. The four main components of PE are: education about trauma and the PE treatment model, breathing exercises (tools to relieve stress and anxiety), in vivo or real world practice with related situations, and imaginal exposure (the repeated talking through of the trauma with a clinician). In this model, it is the repeated exposure that is thought to give the client greater control over unwanted thoughts, feelings, and behaviors, related to the traumatic event (Simpson, 2013, p. 14). This therapy helps people face and control their fear by exposing them to the trauma they experienced in a safe way. It uses mental imagery, writing, or visits to the place where the event happened. The therapist uses these tools to help people with PTSD cope with their feelings. In virtual reality treatment, the person with PTSD is expsoed to a virtual environment that contains the feared situation, instead of taking the person into the actual environment or having the person imagine the traumatic situation. These virtual treatments (computer-based programs) are custom developed to support exposure therapy of anxiety disorders. (ADAA, 2013).

Eye Movement Desensitization and Reprocessing (EMDR): In additiion to cognitive behavioral therapies, EMDR is recommended in most practice guidelines. It involves elements of exposure to traumatic stimuli via imaging and cognitive-behavioral therapy. It may facilitate the accessing and processing traumatic material (Shapiro, 2002). People receiving EMDR engage in imaginal exposure to a trauma while simultaneously performing saccadic eye movements usually by having them follow a wand or other tool with their eyes back and forth. There is good evidence that EMDR is more effective than waitlist and other comparison conditions. Some studies have suggested that eye movements are an unnecessary component and the real power in EMDR is the exposure component (Davidson & Parker, 2001). EMDR is a treatment model that integrates elements from psychodynamic, cognitive behavioral, interpersonal, experiential, and body-centered therapies, which have been found to be effective in the treatment of tauma. It is an information-processing therapy that includes: history-taking, asessment of coping skills and client stability, providing stress reduction tools, identifying a target or current situation which evokes traumatic memory, the use of specific protocols to lessen the intensity of traumatic sensations and increase positive experiences needed for future adaptive behaviors and mental health, and the evaluation of progress (Simpson, 2013, p. 14).

Stress Reduction Inoculation Therapy (SIT): This therapy tries to reduce PTSD symptoms by teaching a person how to reduce anxiety. It helps people look at their memories in a healthy way (ADAA, 2013). It is an integrated cognitive-behavioral therapy that is uniquely designed for each client. The three phases of the work include the initial establishment of trust and a collaborative relationship between the client and clinician, encouraging the client to view symptoms as problems to be addressed and solved, through which the client is taught to analyze a problem into small manageable parts, and developing long-term coping skills. By moving away from an overwhelming global experience of the trauma, a client may develop greater confidence and positive experience in incremental steps in order to manage the impact of trauma on his or her life (Simpson, 2013, p. 14).

Complementary Alternative Modalities: While the following have not undergone the rigorous research involved in stating that a treatment earns the title "best practice," many of the following have shown to be anecdotally effective in helping sufferers of PTSD.

1. Group therapy: Talking with a group of people and sharing their stories can help people with PTSD cope with symptoms and build supportive realtionships with others who have had similar experiences (Simpson, 2013, p. 14).

2. Medication: Medication may also be useful when the anxiety and depression are severe and prevent the person from functioning (Kanel, 2015).

3. Psychodynamic therapy: Because a person suffering from PTSD often oscillates between intrusive thoughts of the traumatic event and numbing of and dissociation of the feelings of the event, Gabbard recommends that those working with individuals with PTSD allow for both the withholding of distressing information and gentle encouragement of the memory of the trauma (2000, p. 256). Lindy et al. (1984) recommend supporting areas of adequate functioning and reestablishing the individual's personal integrity. Psychodynamic treatment would also explore any past traumas that may be worsening the PTSD.

4. Long-term therapy: Seeing a clinician over the course of a few years is sometimes needed to help a person open up about the event that she or he has spent years trying to forget. The longer a victim waits to seek help, the longer the treatment will be. The PTSD sufferer has learned coping skills to survive that may hinder social relationships, work and academic functioning, and her ability to feel spontaneous joy and comfort in the world. Long-term work can offer the person new ways of coping and help him or her understand that the previous defenses that were necessary at one point, are no longer useful.

5. Marital and family therapy: Because family members and spouses are often affected by the unpredictable and often times aggressive behaviors of their loved one suffering from PTSD, working with the entire family may be vital in the overall successful treatment of PTSD. Counselors can support the families of military members during all phases of deployment and help families prepare and adjust (Simpson, 2013, p. 14). Family violence must be dealt with and everyone should be educated on PTSD. Many family members may also be suffering from secondary traumatization (to be discussed below).

PTSD Assessment and Treatment in Older Adults: Kaiser, et al.(2013) propose that age-related factors can interact with posttraumatic stress symptoms and associated problems and carry implications for research and clinical care. Health care professionals need to be well-informed regarding appropriate interventions based on a person's age as well as the broader context of the aging process. They discuss both assessment considerations and treatment considerations when working with older adults suffering from PTSD.

1. <u>Assessment Considerations</u>: A full Mental Status Examination, including a cognitive screening, is recommended by the 2010 VA/DoD Clinical Practice Guideline for PTSD when assessing elderly patients. While most older adults do not have cognitive impairment, an older person who is inattentive to appearance, a poor historian, or forgetful during the interview should be screened for cognitive impairments using standardized instruments. If dementia is suspected the person should be referred for a comprehensive diagnostic evaluation. If delirium is suspected or if there are questions about medication interactions, the person should be referred for medical evaluation. Clinicians should also keep in mind that older clients may not spontaneously report traumatic experiences or they may minimize their importance especially if the event occurred a long time ago. Additionally, older clients may talk about problems or respond to questions differently than younger people. They may be more likely to use general terms like stress and describe emotional difficulties like depression or anxiety as issues or concerns rather than problems. They may present their issues to a primary care clinic rather than seek mental health services. Finally, suicide assessment is particularly important in older clients. For example, older veterans are at greater risk for completed suicide than are middle-aged veterans.

2. <u>Treatment Considerations</u>: There is no evidence that older clients with PTSD cannot benefit from Cognitive Processing Therapy and Prolonged Exposure Therapy or that modifications to the treatment protocols are universally necessary due to older age. However, counselors should consider significant cardiac or respiratory problems because trauma-focused techniques may lead to increased autonomic arousal. These techniques may also lead to decreased cognitive performance and if the older PTSD client already struggles with any cognitive decline, the clinician may need to repeat material, present information in various ways, and focus on one topic at a time. Additionally, counselors may want to engage caregivers in treatment to provide additional support to the client and reinforce the treatment.

Compassion Fatigue/Secondary Traumatization

People who regularly work with individuals in crisis situations may be prone to develop symptoms of PTSD. This phenomenon has been referred to as compassion fatigue, secondary

PTSD, and secondary traumatization. While burnout occurs in many professions, this type of burnout is unique to those who work with survivors of trauma. Symptoms include lack of focus, apathy, rigidity, preoccupation with trauma, anxiety, guilt, anger, numbness, fear, helplessness, sadness, blunted or enhanced affect, irritability, poor sleep, nightmares, appetite change, hypervigilance, isolation, pervasive hopelessness, loss of purpose, skepticism, or loss of faith. When a clinician experiences these symptoms, it is a signal that it's time for a change of pace. It may be time to get away from trauma work for a while, engage in self-care or even one's own therapy (Simpson, 2013, p. 15-16).

Summary

PTSD and AST occur when a person experiences a life threatening trauma to either a loved one or to themselves. Although not all people who experience trauma develop PTSD, it is common enough that clinicians have developed best practices in the treatment of it. The DSM-5 has revised its criteria for the diagnosis of PTSD. Both PTSD and AST have been placed in a new section, Trauma and Stress-Related disorders. In the past it was considered an anxiety disorder, but because there are many symptoms besides anxiety, and because the cause is by definition due to an identifiable stressor, it makes sense to have it exist in a category of its own. There are a variety of stressors that may lead to PTSD, with the biggest stressor being the unexpected, violent loss of a loved one. Military combat, personal victimization, manmade disasters, and natural disasters also may lead to PTSD. Cognitive behavioral treatments such as cognitive processing, exposure therapy, stress inoculation, and EMDR have been shown to be effective in alleviating PTSD symptoms. Both children and older people may exhibit different symptoms than young adults and middle-aged adults and the clinician should be aware of these differences when assessing and treating them. Finally, clinicians may be at risk for developing secondary PTSD/compassion fatigue when working with PTSD sufferers. It is vital for mental health practitioners and other trauma response workers to engage in self-care regularly and monitor any symptoms they may be developing.

Further Resources

Following is a list of websites that offer much information related to PTSD and trauma:

1. Child Welfare Information Gateway: Promotes the safety, permanency, and well-being of children, youth, and families, including a focus on Treatment and Trauma-Informed Care.

   http:/www.childwelfare.gov/responding/trauma.cfm

2. Gift From Within: Provides PTSD resources for survivors and caregivers.

   http://www.giftfromwithin.org/html/articles.html

3. International Society for the Study of Trauma and Disassociation: Includes self-help, listservs, treatment guidelines, trainings, and other links.

    http://www.isst-d.org/sitemap/horizontal-menus/professionals-links.htm

4. National Center for PTSD: The Center focuses on research and education on the prevention, understanding, and treatment of PTSD.

    http://www.ptsd.va.gov/

5. National Child Traumatic Stress Network: Includes psychological first aid field guide.

    http://www.nctsn.org/sites/default/files/pfa/english/1-psyfirstaid_final_complete_manual.pdf

Practice Activities

1. Talk to someone you know about their feelings after 9/11, the Sandy Hook Elementary shootings, and the Boston Marathon Bombing. Try to assess if they exhibited any symptoms of PTSD then or now. Explore their thoughts about what happened.

2. Engage in a self-relaxation exercise. While in a deeply relaxed state, visualize something traumatic that you have experienced. While in that state, explore your thoughts about the trauma and associated feelings. Try to create new, more realistic thoughts about the event.

3. Think of 10 ways in which a person could engage in self-care.

4. How would you explain Rape Trauma Syndrome, Battered Women's Syndrome and Child Abuse Accommodation syndrome to someone?

5. Buy the DSM-5 and review the many revisions.

References

16th Annual National Center for PTSD Report. Retrieved 09/09/2012 from
http://www.ptsd.va.gov/about/annual-report/annual-report-pdf/ar05.pdf

American Psychiatric Association. (2013). *Diagnostic and statistical manual of mental disorder. (5th ed.).* Washington, DC: Author.

American Red Cross. (2001). Emotional health issues for victims. Retrieved from www.trauma-pages.com/notalone.htm

Anxiety and Depression Association of America. (2013). Posttraumatic Stress Disorder (PTSD). Retrieved 11/14/2013 from http://www.adaa.org/understanding-anxiety/posttraumatic-stress-disorder-ptsd?gclid=Cjf...

Bryant, R. A. (2013). An update of Acute Stress Disorder. *PTSD Research Quarterly, 24,1*, 1-7.

Bryant, R. A., Friedman, M.J., Spiegel, D., Ursano, R., and Strain, J. (2011). A review of acute stress disorder in DSM-5. *Depression and Anxiety, 28*, 802-817.

Bryant, R. A., Mastrodomenico, J., Felmingham, K.L., Hopwood, S., Kenny, L., Kandris, E., et al. (2008). Treatment of acute stress disorder: A randomized controlled trial. *Archives of General Psychiatry, 65*, 659-667.

Davidson, P. R., & Parker, K. D. H. (2001). Eye movement desensitization and reprocessing (EMDR): A meta-analysis. *Journal of consulting and clinical psychology, 69*, 305-316.

Department of Veterans Affairs. (2012). National Center for PTSD. How Cognitive Processing Therapy can help. Retrieved 8/30-2012 from http://www.ptsd.va.gov/public/pages/cognitive_processing_therapy.asp

Department of Veteran Affairs. Clinical practice guideline for the management of Post-Traumatic Stress. Retrieved 9/12/2012 from http://www.healthquality.va.gov/ptsd/ptsd_full.pdf

Ehlers, A. and Clark, D. M. (2000). A cognitive model of posttraumatic stress disorder. Behavioral Research and Therapy, 38, 319-345.

Fighting PTSD (20130. Physiological changes in PTSD. Retrieved 11/19/2013 from http://fightingptsd.org/2012/05/19/physiological-changes-in-ptsd/

Fishman, J. (2013). What are some of the physiological manifestations of PTSD? Retrieved 11/19/2013 from

http://psychcentral.com/blog/archives/2013/06/28/what-are-some-of-the-
physiological-m...

Gabbard, G. O. (2000). *Psychodynamic psychiatry in clinical practice (3rd ed.).* Washington,
DC: American Psychiatric Press Inc.

Hamblen, Schnurr, Rosenberg, & Eftekhari. (2013). Overview of Psychotherapy for
PTSD. PTSD: National Center for PTSD. Retrieved 11/14/2013 from
http://www.ptsd.va.gov/professional/pages/overview-treatment-research.asp

Heise, L., Ellsberg, M., & Gottemoeller, M. (1999). Ending violence against women. *Population Reports* (Series L, No. 11). Baltimore: Population Information Program of the Johns
Hopkins University School of Public Health. Volume XXVII, Number 4 December, 1999

Horowitz, M. J. (1976). *Stress Response Syndromes.* New York, Jason Aronson.

Kaiser, A. P., Wachen, J. S., Potter, C., Moye, J., Davison, E., & Hermann, B. (2013).
PTSD Assessment and Treatment in Older Adults. PTSD: National Center for
PTSD. Retrieved 11/14/2013 from
http://www.ptsd.va.gov/professional/pages/assessment_tx_older_adults.asp

Kanel, K. (2015). *A Guide to Crisis Intervention, 5th Ed.* Pacific Grove, CA: Cengage.

Krystal, H. (1988*). Integration and self-healing: Affect, trauma, alexithymia.* Hillsdale,
NJ: Analytic Press.

Ladrech, J. (2004). Serving on CAMFT's Trauma Response Network. *The Therapist, 16,*
6, 20-21.

Lindy, J. D., Grace, M. D.,& Green, B.L. (1984). *Building a conceptual bridge between
civilian trauma and war trauma: preliminary psychological findings from a
clinical sample of Vietnam veterans, in Post-Traumatic Stress Disorder:
Psychological and Biological Sequelae.* Edited by van der Kolk, B. A.,
Washington, DC, American Psychiatric Press, p. 43-57.

Mental Health Center of North Iowa (2005). Background phases of disaster [Online].
Mason City, IA: Author. Available at www.mhconi.org/Topic-disasterBkgrd.htm

Safe Horizon. (2013). Domestic Violence: Statistics and Facts.
http://www.safehorizon.org/index/what-we-do-2/domestic-violence--abuse-53/domestic-
vi... Retrieved 6/19/2013

Shapiro, F. (2002). EMDR twelve years after its introduction: Past and future research. *Journal of Clinical Psychology, 58*: 1-22.

Simpson, P. (2012). Reclaiming Hope: Understanding, treatment, and Resources for clients with PTSD and the clinicians who serve them. *The Therapist, Nov./Dec., Volume 24,* Issue 6, p. 12-16.

Spiegel, D., Koopman, C., Cardena, E., and Classen, C. (1996). Dissociative symptoms in the diagnosis of acute stress disorder. In L. K. Michelson and W. J. Ray (Eds.). *Handbook of dissociation: Empirical, theoretical, and clinical perspective* (pp. 367-380), New York: Plenum.

U.S. Department of Veterans Affairs. (2013). DSM-5 Diagnostic Criteria for PTSD Released. Retrieved 11/14/2013 from

http://www.ptsd.va.gov/professional/pages/diagnostic_criteria_dsm-5.asp

Yarvis, J. S. (2013). Posttraumatic Stress disorder (PTSD) in Veterans. Found in the *Handbook of Military Social Work,* Edited by Rubin, A., Weiss, E. L. & Coll, J. E. John New Jersey: Wiley & Sons, Inc. p. 81-97.

U.S. Bureau of Justice. (2013). Rape Statistics. http://www.statisticbrain.com/rape-statistics/ Retrieved 10/23/2013.

U. S. Bureau of Justice. (2013). Female Victims of Sexual Violence, 1994-2010. http://www.bjs.gov/index.cfm?ty=pbdetail&iid-4594 Retrieved 10/23/2010.

Walker, J. (2001). The relevance of shame in child protection work. *Journal of Social Work Practice, 6,* 4, 451-463.

Walker, L. E. A. (1984). *Battered Woman Syndrome.* New York: Springer Publishing.

NOTES

NOTES

NOTES

NOTES

NOTES

NOTES

NOTES

NOTES

NOTES

NOTES